THE ULTIMATE

KETO DIET

COOKBOOK

FOR BEGINNERS

Live Healthier and Lose Weight Easily with The Best Low
Carb High Fat Recipes!

GRACELYNN ROGERS

MARY J. GREEN

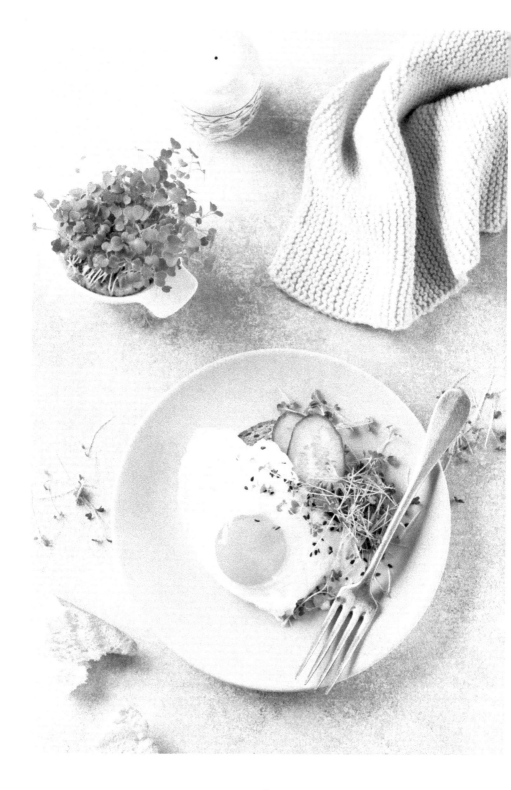

TABLE OF CONTENTS

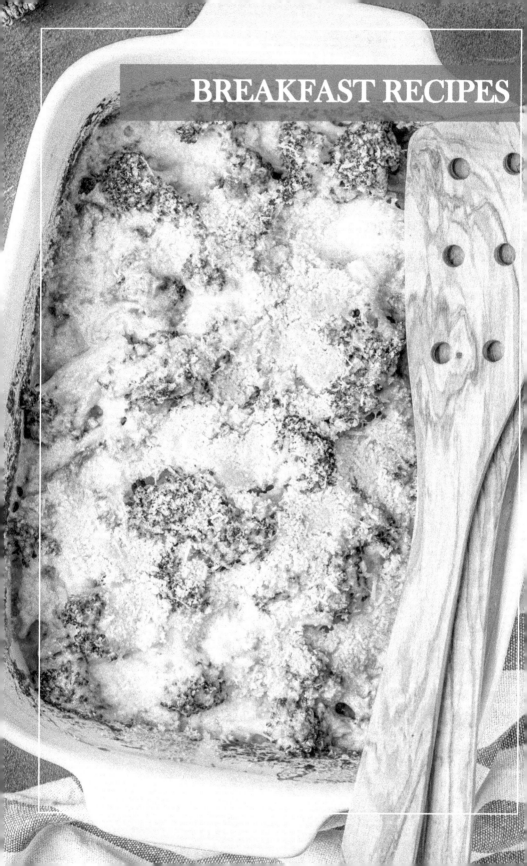

NUTTY TEXTURED PORRIDGE

Prep time: 15 min
Cook time: 35 min
Servings: 05

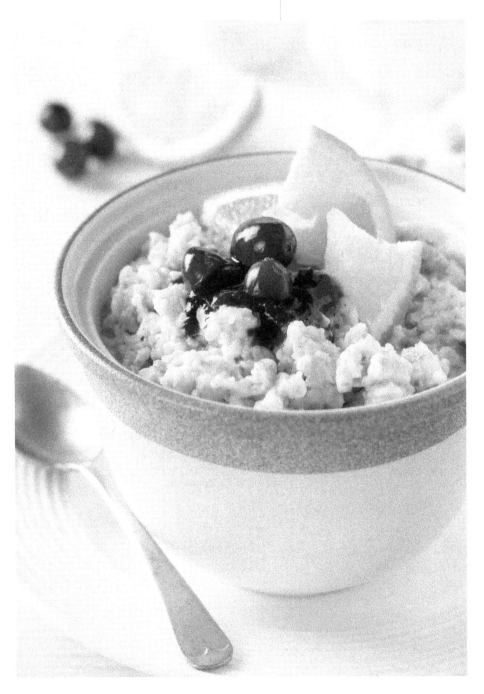

Ingredients

½ cup pecans

½ cup walnuts

¼ cup sunflower seeds

¼ cup chia seeds

¼ cup unsweetened coconut flakes

4 cups unsweetened almond milk

½ tsp. ground cinnamon

¼ tsp. ground ginger

1 tsp. stevia powder

1 tbsp. butter.

Directions

1. In a food processor, place the pecans, walnuts and sunflower seeds and pulse until a crumbly mixture is formed.

2. In a large pan, add the nuts mixture, chia seeds, coconut flakes, almond milk, spices and stevia powder over medium heat and bring to a gentle simmer, stirring frequently.

3. Select heat to low and simmer for about 20-30 minutes, stirring frequently.

4. Remove from the heat and serve hot with the topping of butter.

Nutrition

Calories 269 kcal | Carbs: 8.6g | Protein: 7g.

PEAR & PEANUT BUTTER SMOOTHIE

Prep time: 10 min

Cook time: 0 min

Servings: 01

Ingredients

1 pear, peeled, cored
and chopped

¾ cup unsweetened
almond milk

½ tbsp. smooth peanut
butter

½ tsp. fresh ginger,
grated

¼ tsp. ground cinnamon

A handful of ice.

Directions

1. In a high-speed blender, combine all of
   the ingredients.

2. Blend until smooth, then transfer into
   a tall glasse filled with ice.

3. Top with pear and cinnamon crisps to
   serve (optional).

Nutrition

Calories 163 kcal | Fat: 5.5g | Carbs: 2g |
Protein: 3.1g.

CHOCOLATE CHIA PUDDING

Prep time: 1 h 5 min

Cook time: 0 min

Servings: 04

Ingredients

½ cup black chia seeds

2 tbsp. unsweetened cocoa powder

4 tbsp. stevia

2 cups unsweetened almond milk

2 tsp. vanilla extract.

For Topping (optional)

Coconut yogurt

Seasonal fruit, sliced

Directions

1. In a large mixing bowl, combine chia seeds, sifted cocoa powder, and stevia. Stir well to remove any lumps.

2. Then add in the almond milk and vanilla extract and whisk until well combined.

3. Cover and refrigerate overnight (or for at least 1 hour).

4. Dish up the chocolate chia pudding right before serving. Add coconut yogurt and seasonal fruit. Enjoy!

Nutrition

Calories 335 kcal | Fat: 26.9g | Carbs: 15g | Protein: 8.2g.

KETO MUFFINS

Prep time: 10 min
Cook time: 23 min
Servings: 06

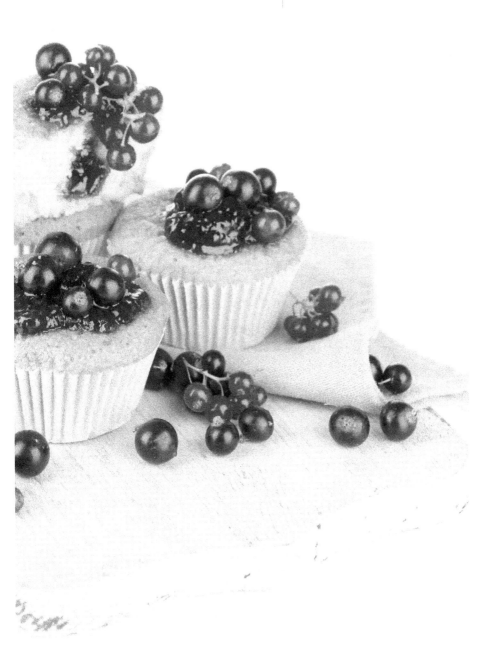

Ingredients

2 cups almond flour

½ cup powdered Swerve

3 scoops turmeric tonic

1½ tsp. organic baking powder

3 organic eggs

1 cup mayonnaise

½ tsp. organic vanilla extract.

Directions

1. Ready the oven to 350°F. Line a 12 cups muffin tin with paper liners.

2. In a large bowl, add the flour, Swerve, turmeric tonic and baking powder and mix well.

3. Add the eggs, mayonnaise and vanilla extract and beat until well combined. Place the mixture into the prepared muffin cups evenly. Bake for about 20-23 minutes.

4. Pull out the muffin tin. Position onto the wire rack to cool for 8 minutes.

5. Carefully invert the muffins onto the wire rack to cool completely before serving.

Nutrition

Calories 489 | Carbs: 9.5g | Protein: 10.8g.

BLUEBERRY WAFFLES

Prep time: 11 min

Cook time: 17 min

Servings: 09

Ingredients

8 eggs

5 oz. melted butter

1 tsp. vanilla extract

2 tsp. baking powder

⅓ cup coconut flour.

Topping:

3 oz. butter

1 oz. fresh blueberries.

Directions

1. Start by mixing the butter and eggs first until you get a smooth batter. Put in the remaining ingredients except those that you will be using as topping.

2. Heat your waffle iron to medium temperature and start pouring in the batter for cooking.

3. In a separate bowl, mix the butter and blueberries using a hand mixer. Use this to top off your freshly cooked waffles.

Nutrition

Calories 575 kcal| Fat 56g | Carbs: 15g | Fiber 5g | Protein: 36g.

KETO PANCAKES

Ingredients

½ cup almond flour

4 oz. cream cheese, softened

4 large organic eggs

1 tsp. lemon zest

Butter, for frying and serving.

Directions

1. In a medium bowl, whisk together almond flour, cream cheese, eggs, and lemon zest until smooth.

2. In a nonstick skillet over medium-low heat, melt 1 tablespoon butter. Pour in about 3 tablespoons batter and cook until golden, 2 minutes.

3. Flip and cook 2 minutes more. Transfer to a plate and repeat with remaining batter.

4. You can serve it topped with butter and fresh berries. Enjoy!

Nutrition

Calories 110 kcal | Fat: 3.5g | Carbs: 2g | Protein: 4g.

JALAPENO POPPER EGG CUPS

Prep time: 5 min

Cook time: 15 min

Servings: 06

Ingredients

5 large eggs

¾ tsp. salt

¼ tsp. black pepper

½ tsp. onion powder

½ tsp. garlic powder

½ cup Cheddar cheese, grated

⅓ cup cream cheese, softened

3-4 Jalapeno peppers, de-seeded and chopped

⅓ cup bacon, cooked crumbled.

Directions

1. Preheat the oven to 400°F and grease muffin tray with cooking spray. Set aside.

2. In a medium mixing bowl, whisk together eggs, onion powder, garlic powder, cream cheese, salt and pepper.

3. Stir in Cheddar cheese, chopped jalapeno peppers, and crumbled bacon. Mix until well combined.

4. Divide the mixture evenly into 6 muffin cups, filling each about 2/3 full.

5. Bake for about 12-15 minutes.

6. Serve hot.

Nutrition

Calories 120 kcal | Fat: 4g | Carbs: 1.4g | Protein: 5g.

SAVORY CHEDDAR OMELET

Ingredients

4 large eggs

2 oz. cheddar cheese, shredded

8 olives, pitted

2 tbsp. butter

2 tbsp. olive oil

1 tsp. herb de Provence

½ tsp. salt.

Directions

1. Whisk eggs in a bowl with salt, olives, herb de Provence, and olive oil.

2. Melt butter in a large pan over medium heat.

3. Pour egg mixture into the hot pan and spread evenly.

4. Cover and cook for 3 minutes or until omelet lightly golden brown.

5. Flip omelet to the other side and cook for 2 minutes more.

6. Serve and enjoy!

Nutrition

Calories 251 kcal | Fat: 22g | Carbs 1.1g.

SPINACH & FETA BREAKFAST WRAPS

Ingredients

1 tsp. olive oil

½ cup fresh baby spinach leaves

1 tbsp. fresh basil

4 egg whites, beaten

½ tsp. salt

¼ tsp. freshly ground black pepper

¼ cup crumbled low-fat feta cheese

2 (8-inch) whole-wheat tortillas.

Directions

1. Heat up olive oil on medium heat. Sauté spinach and basil to the pan for about 2 minutes.

2. Add the egg whites to the pan, season with the salt and pepper, and sauté, often stirring, for about 2 minutes more, or until the egg whites are firm.

3. Remove from the heat and sprinkle with the feta cheese.

4. Warm up tortillas in the microwave for 20 to 30 seconds. Divide the eggs between the tortillas and wrap up burrito-style.

Nutrition

Calories 224 kcal | Fat: 10.4g | Carbs: 4.5g | Protein: 10.6g.

AVOCADO TOASTS WITH 3 TOPPINGS

Prep time: 20 min
Cook time: 45 min
Servings: 03

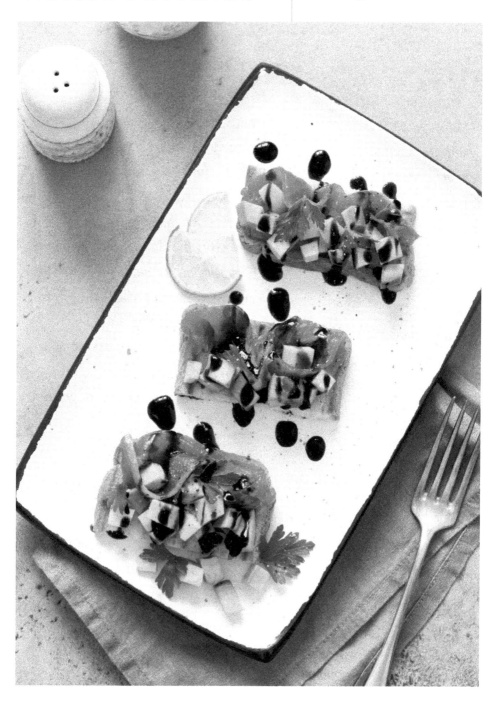

Ingredients

Directions

Keto Seed Crackers:

1½ tbsp. almond flour

1½ tbsp. unsalted sunflower seeds

1½ tbsp. unsalted pumpkin seeds

1½ tbsp. flaxseed or chia seeds

1½ tbsp. sesame seeds

½ tbsp. ground psyllium husk powder

½ tsp. salt

1¼ tbsp. melted coconut oil

½ cup. boiling water.

Keto Seed Crackers:

1. Preheat the oven to 300°F.

2. Mix all dry ingredients in a bowl. Add boiling water and oil. Mix together well.

3. Keep working the dough until it forms a ball and has a gel-like consistency.

4. Place the dough on a baking sheet lined with parchment paper. Add another paper on top and use a rolling pin to flatten the dough evenly.

5. Remove the upper paper and bake on the lower rack for about 40-45 minutes, check occasionally. Seeds are heat sensitive so pay close attention towards the end.

6. Turn off the oven and leave the crackers to dry in the oven. Once dried and cool, break into 9 equal pieces and spread a generous amount of butter on top.

Toppings:

3 ripe avocados

3 lime3 (or lemon3)

Avocado Toasts:

7. Slice avocados lengthwise. Remove the seeds and the skin. Mash or slice

Black pepper and sea salt, to taste

Fresh chili pepper, to taste

3 softly boiled or poached eggs

3 handfuls Romaine lettuce

3 pinches of parsley

6 fin slices of smoked (wild) salmon

3 handfuls mixed lettuce

3 pinches of dill.

avocados. Season with lime or lemon juice, black pepper and sea salt.

8. Top all the seed crackers with avocado.

9. Version 1: top 3 crackers with finely sliced chili pepper (seeds removed).

10. Version 2: top other 3 crackers with a softly boiled or poached eggs, finely chopped parsley and shredded Romaine lettuce.

11. Version 3: top last 3 crackers with smoked salmon, dill and mixed young lettuce leaves.

12. Enjoy!

Nutrition

Calories 224 kcal | Fat: 10.4g | Carbs: 4.5g | Protein: 10.6g.

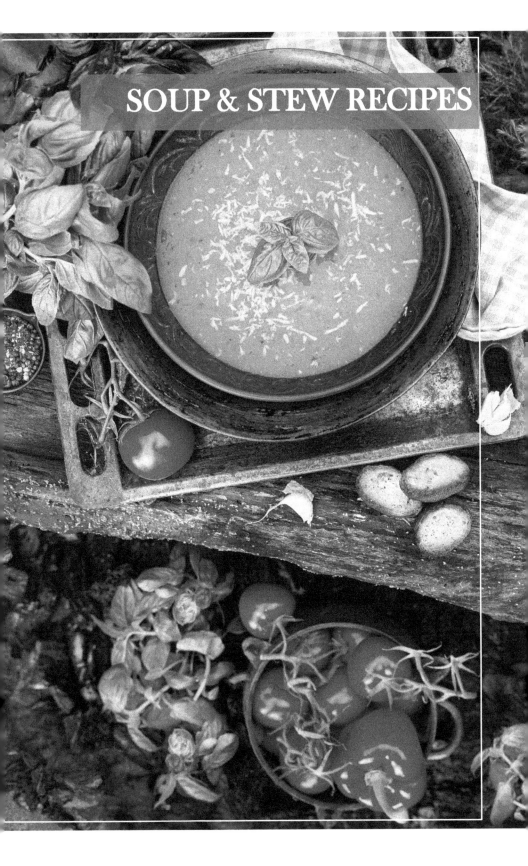

SOUP & STEW RECIPES

EASY SUMMER GAZPACHO

Prep time: 1h 10 min

Cook time: 0 min

Servings: 06

Ingredients

4 medium tomatoes chopped

1 English cucumber, peeled and chopped

¼ medium red onion, chopped

⅓ cup fresh parsley, chopped

12 fresh basil leaves

1 lemon juice

1 tbsp. extra-virgin olive oil

Salt and black pepper, to taste

½ cup grape tomatoes, quartered.

Directions

1. In a high-speed blender, combine all of the ingredients (except grape tomatoes), leaving apart ¼ of chopped cucumber, ¼ of chopped onion, ¼ of chopped parsley and 4 basil leaves.

2. Blend until smooth and creamy or about 2 minutes,

3. Then transfer into a large container, add in remaining chopped vegetables, cover and chill for 1 hour.

4. When ready to serve, divide the soup among 6 bowls and garnish with remaining herbs

Nutrition

Calories 92 kcal | Fat: 1.5g | Carbs: 10g | Protein: 2.3g.

FRESH AVOCADO SOUP

Prep time: 5 min

Cook time: 10 min

Servings: 02

Ingredients

1 ripe avocado

2 romaine lettuce leaves

1 cup coconut milk, chilled

1 tbsp. lime juice

20 fresh mint leaves.

Directions

1. Mix all your ingredients thoroughly in a blender.

2. Chill in the fridge for 5-10 minutes before serving.

Nutrition

Calories 280 kcal | Fat: 26g | Carbs: 2.6g | Protein: 4g

COLD ITALIAN CUCUMBER SOUP

Prep time: 2h 10min
Cook time: 0 min
Servings: 04

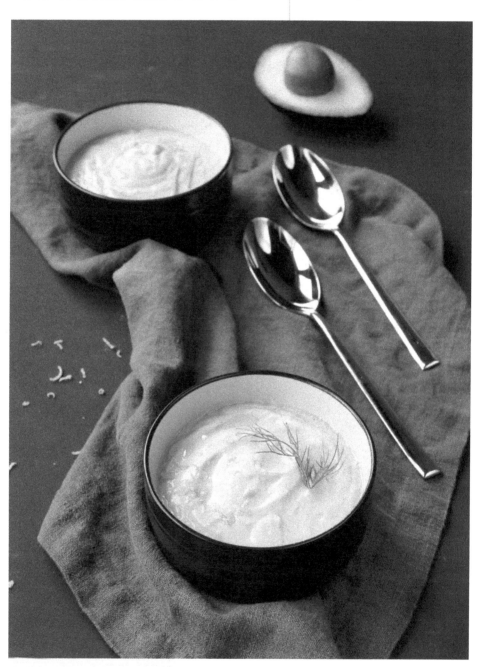

Ingredients   **Directions**

3 cucumbers, chopped

2 ripe avocados, peeled and pitted

2 spring onions, chopped

2 garlic cloves, minced

5 fresh basil leaves

2 tbsp. fresh parsley, chopped

2 cups vegetable stock

3 tbsp. lime juice

¼ cup extra virgin olive oil

Salt and black pepper, to taste.

For Topping

3 tbsp. extra virgin olive oil

1 cucumber, thinly sliced

4 fresh basil leaves

4 dried tomatoes

8 little mozzarellas, halved

1. In a high-speed blender combine chopped cucumbers, vegetable stock, avocado halves, lime juice, chopped onions, minced garlic cloves, basil leaves, and chopped parsley.

2. Process for 2-3 minutes, until smooth and creamy.

3. Transfer the soup into a container, cover and refrigerate for at least 2 hours before serving.

4. When ready to serve, pour the creamy chilled soup into 2 serving plates.

5. Top with the extra virgin olive oil, cucumber slices, basil leaves, dried tomatoes, and mozzarella halves.

6. Season with salt and pepper. Enjoy!

Nutrition

Calories 317 kcal | Fat: 25g | Carbs: 4.7g | Protein: 6g.

TOMATO SOUP & GRILLED CHEESE SANDWICHES

Prep time: 18 min

Cook time: 40 min

Servings: 04

Ingredients

3 tbsp. unsalted butter

1 tbsp. almond oil

1 (7 oz.) cans crushed tomatoes

2 medium white onions

1½ cups water

Salt and black pepper, to taste

1 tsp. dried basil

8 low-carb bread slices

1 cup Gruyere cheese

½ cup grated Monterey Jack cheese

1 tbsp. chopped fresh basil for garnish.

Directions

1. Cook 2 tablespoons of butter in a pot and mix in the tomatoes, onions, and water.

2. Season with salt, black pepper, basil, and bring the mixture to a boil.

3. Reduce the heat immediately and simmer for 30 minutes or until the liquid reduces by a third.

4. Meanwhile, melt a ¼ tablespoon of butter in a non-stick skillet over medium heat and lay in a bread slice.

5. Add a quarter each of both cheese on top and cover with another bread slice.

6. Once the cheese starts melting and beneath the bread is golden brown, about 1 minute, flip the sandwich.

7. Cook further for 1 more minute or until the other side of the bread is golden brown too.

8. Remove the sandwich to a plate and make three more in the same manner.

9. Afterwards, diagonally slice each sandwich in half.

10. Dish the tomato soup into serving bowls when ready, garnish with the basil leaves, and serve warm with the sandwiches.

Nutrition

Calories 285 kcal | Fat: 25.2g | Carbs: 13g | Protein: 12g.

CREAMY TAHINI ZOODLE SOUP

Prep time: 15min

Cook time: 14 min

Servings: 04

Ingredients

2 tbsp. coconut oil

2 tbsp. butter

½ medium onion, chopped

½ cup sliced cremini mushrooms

1 garlic clove, minced

4 cups vegetable broth

4 tbsp. coconut aminos

2 tbsp. erythritol

2 tbsp. tahini

4 tbsp. heavy cream

4 zucchinis, spiralized.

For Topping

1 tbsp. toasted sesame oil

1 tbsp. chopped fresh scallions

1 tbsp. toasted sesame seeds.

Directions

1. Warm up coconut oil and butter in a pot.

2. Stir-fry the onion, and mushrooms for 5 minutes or until softened.

3. Mix in the garlic and cook for 30 seconds or until fragrant.

4. Add the vegetable broth, coconut aminos, erythritol, tahini, heavy cream, and stir well. Boil the mix then, simmer for 5 minutes.

5. Mix in the zucchinis and cook for 3 minutes or until the zucchinis are tender.

6. Drizzle with the sesame oil, scallions, and sesame seeds.

Nutrition

Calories 347 kcal | Fat: 36g | Carbs: 6.5g | Protein: 11g.

GREEK EGG LEMON CHICKEN SOUP

Prep time: 5 min

Cook time: 30 min

Servings: 04

Ingredients

4 cups of water

¾ lb. cauli

1 lb. boneless chicken thighs

⅓ lb. butter

4 eggs

1 lemon

2 tbsps. fresh parsley

1 bay leaf

2 chicken bouillon cubes

Salt and pepper.

Directions

1. Slice your chicken thinly and then place it in a saucepan while adding cold water and the cubes and bay leaf. Let the meat simmer for 10 mins before removing it and the bay leaf.

2. Grate your cauli and place it in a saucepan. Add butter and boil for a few minutes.

3. Beat your eggs and lemon juice in a bowl, while seasoning it.

4. Reduce the heat a bit and add the eggs, stirring continuously. Let simmer but don't boil.

5. Return in the chicken.

Nutrition

Calories 582 kcal | Fat: 49g | Carbs: 7.1g | Protein: 31g.

CAULIFLOWER RICE & CHICKEN SOUP

Prep time: 10 min

Cook time: 1 h

Servings: 05

Ingredients

2½ lb. chicken breasts

8 tbsp. butter

¼ cup celery, chopped

½ cup onion, chopped

4 cloves garlic, minced

2 (12-oz) packages steamed cauliflower rice

1 tbsp. parsley

2 tsp. poultry seasoning

½ cup carrot, grated

¾ tsp. rosemary

Salt and pepper

4 oz. cream cheese

4¾ cup chicken broth.

Directions

1. Put shredded chicken breasts into a saucepan and pour in the chicken broth. Add salt and pepper. Cook for 1 hour.

2. In another pot, melt the butter. Add the onion, garlic, and celery. Sauté until the mix is translucent. Add the rice cauliflower, rosemary, and carrot. Mix and cook for 7 minutes.

3. Mix chicken breasts and broth to the cauliflower mix. Put the lid on and simmer for 15 minutes.

Nutrition

Calories 415 kcal | Fat: 30g | Carbs: 9.8g | Protein: 27g

ASPARAGUS PUREE SOUP

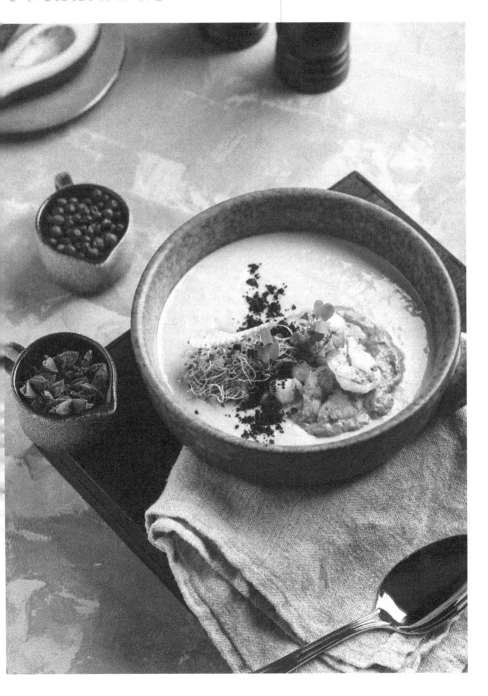

Ingredients

2 tbsp. butter

1 garlic clove, minced

2 lb. asparagus, ends
trimmed, cut into 1"
pieces

2 cup low-sodium
chicken broth

½ cup heavy cream

Salt and black pepper,
to taste.

For Garnish

4 tbsp. heavy cream

4 tbsp. fresh chives,
chopped

4 tbsp. fresh dill,
chopped.

Directions

1. In a heavy pot over medium heat, melt butter. Add garlic and sauté for 1 minute.

2. Add asparagus and cook for about 5 minutes, until golden.

3. Add broth and simmer, covered for 10 to 15 minutes, until asparagus is tender but still green.

4. Puree the soup with an immersion blender. Then stir in heavy cream and warm over low heat. Season with salt and pepper to taste.

5. Dish up the soup, garnish with a spoon of heavy cream, fresh chives, and fresh dill. Serve hot.

Nutrition

Calories 246 kcal | Fat: 27g | Carbs: 5.9g | Protein: 10g.

CREAMY CHICKEN POT PIE SOUP

Prep time: 20 min

Cook time: 35 min

Servings: 06

Ingredients

2 tbsp. extra-virgin olive oil, divided

1 lb. skinless chicken breast

1 cup mushrooms, quartered

2 celery stalks, chopped

1 onion, chopped

1 tbsp. garlic, minced

5 cups low-sodium chicken broth

1 cup green beans, chopped

¼ cup cream cheese

1 cup heavy whipping cream

1 tbsp. fresh thyme, chopped.

Directions

1. Cook olive oil in a stockpot over medium-high heat until shimmering.

2. Add the chicken chunks to the pot and sauté for 10 minutes or until well browned.

3. Transfer the chicken to a plate. Set aside until ready to use.

4. Heat the remaining olive oil in the stockpot over medium-high heat.

5. Add the mushrooms, celery, onion, and garlic to the pot and sauté for 6 minutes or until fork-tender.

6. Pour the chicken broth over, then add the cooked chicken chunks to the pot. Stir to mix well and boil the soup. Adjust the heat to low. Simmer the for 15 minutes.

7. Mix in the green beans, cream cheese, cream, thyme, salt, and black pepper, then simmer for 3 more minutes.

8. Remove the soup from the stockpot and serve hot.

Nutrition

Calories 338 kcal | Fat: 26.1g | Carbs: 24g | Protein: 28g.

CHUNKY PORK SOUP

Prep time: 25 min

Cook time: 30 min

Servings: 02

Ingredients

1 tbsp. olive oil

1 bell pepper, deveined and chopped

2 garlic cloves, pressed

½ cup scallions, chopped

½-pound ground pork (84% lean)

1 cup beef bone broth

1 cup of water

½ tsp. crushed red pepper flakes

1 bay laurel

1 tsp. fish sauce

2 cups mustard greens, torn into pieces

1 tbsp. fresh parsley, chopped.

Directions

1. Coat, once hot, sauté the pepper, garlic, and scallions until tender or about 3 minutes.

2. After that, stir in the ground pork and cook for 5 minutes more or until well browned, stirring periodically.

3. Add in the beef bone broth, water, red pepper, salt, black pepper, and bay laurel. Reduce the temperature to simmer and cook, covered, for 10 minutes. Afterward, stir in the fish sauce and mustard greens.

4. Remove from the heat; let it stand until the greens are wilted.

5. Ladle into individual bowls and serve garnished with fresh parsley.

Nutrition

Calories 344 kcal | Fat: 25.2g | Carbs: 12.1g | Protein: 23.1g.

CABBAGE SOUP WITH BEEF

Prep time: 15 min

Cook time: 20 min

Servings: 04

Ingredients

2 tbsp. olive oil

1 medium onion, chopped

1-pound fillet steak, cut into pieces

½ stalk celery, chopped

1 carrot, peeled and diced

½ head small green cabbage

2 cloves garlic, minced

4 cups beef broth

2 tbsp. fresh parsley, chopped

1 tsp. thyme, dried

1 tsp. rosemary, dried

1 tsp. garlic powder.

Directions

1. Heat oil in a pot (use medium heat). Add the beef and cook until it is browned. Put the onion into the pot and boil for 3-4 minutes.

2. Add the celery and carrot. Stir well and cook for about 3-4 minutes. Add the cabbage and boil until it starts softening. Add garlic and simmer for about 1 minute.

3. Pour the broth into the pot. Add the parsley and garlic powder. Mix thoroughly and reduce heat to medium-low.

4. Cook for 10-15 minutes.

Nutrition

Calories 177 kcal | Fat: 11g | Carbs: 3g | Protein: 12g.

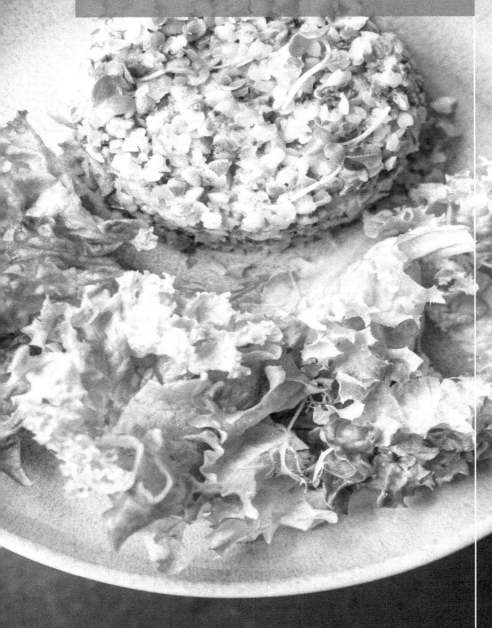

CITRUS EGG SALAD

Prep time: 10 min

Cook time: 20 min

Servings: 03

Ingredients

6 eggs

1 tsp. Dijon mustard

2 tbsp. of mayo

1 tsp. of lemon juice.

Directions

1. Place the eggs gently in a medium saucepan.
2. Add cold water until your eggs are covered by an inch.
3. Bring to a boil.
4. You should do this for ten minutes. Remove from your heat and cool. Peel your eggs under running water that is cold.
5. Put your eggs in a food processor. Pulse until they are chopped.
6. Stir in condiments and juice.

Nutrition

Calories 22 kcal | Fat: 19g | Carbs: 8g | Protein: 13g.

TOMATO & MOZZA SALAD

Prep time: 15 min

Cook time: 10 min

Servings: 08

Ingredients

4 cups cherry tomatoes

1½ lb. mozzarella cheese

¼ cup fresh basil leaves

¼ cup olive oil

2 tbsp. fresh lemon juice

1 tsp. fresh oregano

1 tsp. fresh parsley

3 drops liquid stevia.

Directions

1. In a salad bowl, mix together tomatoes, mozzarella, and basil.
2. In a small bowl, add remaining ingredients and beat until well combined.
3. Place dressing over salad and toss to coat well.
4. Serve immediately.

Nutrition

Calories 87 kcal | Fat: 7.5g | Carbs: 5.2g | Protein: 2.4g.

SHRIMP LETTUCE WRAPS WITH BUFFALO SAUCE

Prep time: 15 min

Cook time: 20 min

Servings: 04

Ingredients

1 egg, beaten

3 tbsp. butter

16 oz. shrimp, peeled, deveined, with tails removed

¾ cup almond flour

¼ cup hot sauce (like Frank's)

1 tsp. extra-virgin olive oil

1 head romaine lettuce, leaves parted, for serving

½ red onion, chopped

Celery, finely sliced

½ blue cheese, cut into pieces.

Directions

1. To make the Buffalo sauce, melt the butter in a saucepan, add the garlic and cook this mixture for 1 minute. Pour hot sauce into the saucepan and whisk to combine. Set aside.

2. In one bowl, crack one egg, add salt and pepper and mix. In another bowl, put the almond flour, add salt and pepper and also combine. Dip each shrimp into the egg mixture first and then into the almond one.

3. Take a large frying pan. Heat the oil and cook your shrimp for about 2 minutes per side.

4. Add Buffalo sauce.

5. Serve in lettuce leaves. Top your shrimp with red onion, blue cheese, and celery.

Nutrition

Calories 213 kcal | Fat: 54g | Carbs: 8g | Protein: 33g.

CREAMY KETO EGG SALAD

Prep time: 5 min

Cook time: 15 min

Servings: 04

Ingredients

8 large eggs, boiled

1/2 cup low carb mayonnaise

1 tbsp. chives, finely chopped

1 tsp. lemon juice

2 tsp. Dijon mustard

½ tsp. salt

¼ tsp. freshly ground black pepper

A pinch of paprika.

Directions

1. Peel and dice the eggs.
2. In a mixing bowl combine all of the ingredients and stir gently.
3. Adjust salt and pepper to taste and serve.

Nutrition

Calories 413 kcal | Fat: 10g | Carbs: 2g | Protein: 12g.

SMOKED SALMON FILLED AVOCADOS

Prep time: 13 min

Cook time: 5 min

Servings: 02

Ingredients

1 medium avocado

3 oz. smoked salmon

4 tbsp. sour cream

1 tbsp. lemon juice

Pepper and salt, to taste.

Directions

1. Cut the avocado into two and discard the pit.

2. Place the same amounts of sour cream in the hollow parts of the avocado. Include smoked salmon on top.

3. Season with pepper and salt, squeeze lemon juice over the top.

Nutrition

Calories 517 kcal | Fats: 42.6g | Carbs: 5.9g | Protein: 20.6g.

MUSHROOM OMELET

Prep time: 10 min

Cook time: 5 min

Servings: 01

Ingredients

3 medium eggs

1 oz. cheese, shredded

1 oz. butter used for frying

¼ yellow onion, chopped

4 large mushrooms, sliced

Your favorite vegetables (optional).

Directions

1. Scourge eggs in a bowl. Add some salt and pepper to taste.

2. Cook butter in a pan using low heat. Put in the mushroom and onion, cooking the two until you get that amazing smell.

3. Pour the egg mix into the pan and allow it to cook on medium heat. Allow the bottom part to cook before sprinkling the cheese on top of the still-raw portion of the egg.

4. Carefully pry the edges of the omelet and fold it in half. Allow it to cook for a few more seconds before removing the pan from the heat and sliding it directly onto your plate.

Nutrition

Calories 520 kcal | Fat: 27g | Carbs: 5g | Protein: 26g.

AVOCADO TACO

Prep time: 10 min

Cook time: 15 min

Servings: 06

Ingredients

1-pound ground beef

3 avocados, halved

1 tbsp. Chili powder

½ tsp. salt

¾ tsp. cumin

½ tsp. oregano, dried

¼ tsp. garlic powder

¼ tsp. onion powder

8 tbsp. tomato sauce

1 cup Cheddar cheese, shredded

¼ cup cherry tomatoes, sliced

¼ cup lettuce, shredded

½ cup sour cream.

Directions

1. Pit halved avocados. Set aside.
2. Place the ground beef into a saucepan. Cook at medium heat until it is browned.
3. Add the seasoning and tomato sauce. Stir well and cook for about 4 minutes.
4. Load each avocado half with the beef.
5. Top with shredded cheese and lettuce, tomato slices, and sour cream.

Nutrition

Calories 278 kcal | Fat: 22g | Carbs: 14g | Protein: 18g.

KETO CAESAR SALAD

Ingredients

1½ cup mayonnaise

3 tbsp. apple cider vinegar/acv

1 tsp. Dijon mustard

4 anchovy filets

24 romaine heart leaves

4 oz. pork rinds, chopped

Parmesan (for garnish).

Directions

1. Place the mayo with ACV, mustard, and anchovies into a blender and process until smooth and dressing like.

2. Prepare romaine leaves and pour out dressing across them evenly. Top with pork rinds and enjoy.

Nutrition

Calories 400 kcal | Fat: 25g | Carbs: 9g | Protein: 33g.

CHICKEN CLUB LETTUCE WRAP

Prep time: 15 min

Cook time: 15 min

Servings: 01

Ingredients

1 head of iceberg
lettuce with the core
and outer leaves
removed

1 tbsp. of mayonnaise

6 slices or organic
chicken or turkey breast

2 cooked strips of
bacon

2 slices tomato

Directions

1. Line your working surface with a large slice of parchment paper. Layer 6-8 large leaves of lettuce in the center of the paper to make a base of around 9-10 inches. Spread the mayo in the center and lay with chicken or turkey, bacon, and tomato.

2. Starting with the end closest to you, roll the wrap like a jelly roll with the parchment paper as your guide. Keep it tight and halfway through, roll tuck in the ends of the wrap.

3. When it is completely wrapped, roll the rest of the parchment paper around it, and use a knife to cut it in half.

Nutrition

Calories 207 kcal | Carbs: 6g | Protein: 12g | Fat: 15g.

SCALLOPS IN GARLIC SAUCE

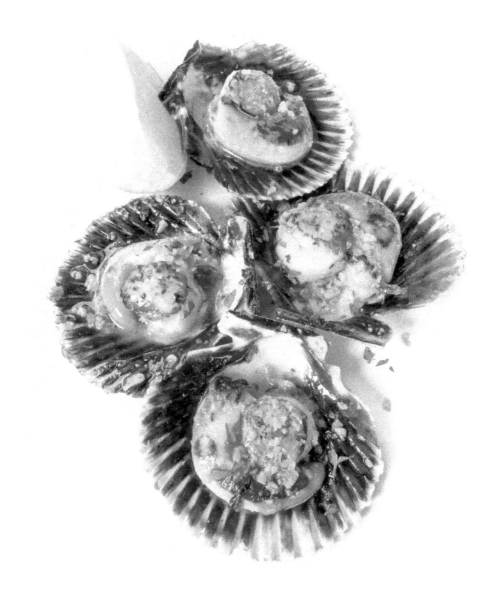

Ingredients

1¼ lb. fresh sea scallops

4 tbsp. butter, divided

5 garlic cloves, chopped

¼ cup homemade chicken broth

1 cup heavy cream

1 tbsp. fresh lemon juice

2 tbsp. fresh parsley.

Directions

1. Sprinkle the scallops evenly with salt and black pepper.

2. Melt 2 tablespoons of butter in a large pan over medium-high heat and cook the scallops for about 2–3 minutes per side.

3. Flip the scallops and cook for about 2 more minutes.

4. With a slotted spoon, transfer the scallops onto a plate.

5. Now, melt the remaining butter in the same pan over medium heat and sauté the garlic for about 1 minute.

6. Pour the broth and bring to a gentle boil. Cook for about 2 minutes. Stir in the cream and cook for about 1–2 minutes or until slightly thickened.

7. Stir in the cooked scallops and lemon juice and remove from heat. Garnish with fresh parsley and serve hot.

Nutrition

Calories 435 kcal | Fat: 33g | Carbs: 12.4g | Protein: 25g.

BUTTER TROUT WITH BOK CHOY

Prep time: 15 min

Cook time: 30 min

Servings: 06

Ingredients

½ tbsp. honey

1 tbsp. tamari

1 large garlic clove

¾ tsp. chili powder

1 filet (6 oz.) trout fish

2 heads baby bok choy

½ tsp. sesame oil

¼ tsp. hot pepper flakes.

Directions

1. Prep oven to 425°F and line a baking sheet with parchment paper.

2. Scourge honey, half the tamari, minced garlic and chili powder.

3. Arrange rainbow trout skin side down onto parchment paper and season. Use a brush to spread the honey garlic mixture onto the fish.

4. Toss bok choy to a large mixing bowl and drizzle with the remaining tamari and sesame oil. Situate bok choy to baking sheet and organize it around the rainbow trout. Bake for 12 to 15 minutes.

Nutrition

Calories 352 kcal | Fat: 37g | Carbs: 2g | Protein: 42.5g.

BUTTER CHICKEN

Prep time: 15 min

Cook time: 30 min

Servings: 05

Ingredients

3 tbsp. unsalted butter

1 medium yellow onion, chopped

2 garlic cloves, minced

1 tsp. fresh ginger, minced

1½ lb. grass-fed chicken breasts

2 tomatoes, chopped finely

1 tbsp. garam masala

1 tsp. red chili powder

1 tsp. ground cumin

1 cup heavy cream

2 tbsp. fresh cilantro.

Directions

1. Cook butter in a large wok over medium-high heat and sauté the onions for about 5–6 minutes. Add in ginger and garlic and sauté for about 1 minute. Add the tomatoes and cook for about 2–3 minutes, crushing with the back of spoon.

2. Stir in the chicken spices, salt, and black pepper, and cook for about 6–8 minutes or until desired doneness of the chicken.

3. Drizzle the heavy cream and cook for about 8–10 more minutes, stirring occasionally. Garnish with fresh cilantro and serve hot.

Nutrition

Calories 507 kcal | Fat: 33g | Carbs: 14g | Protein: 41g.

BACON ROASTED CHICKEN WITH PAN GRAVY

Prep time: 8 min

Cook time: 1h 5 min

Servings: 08

Ingredients

3 lb. whole chicken, gutted

4 sprigs fresh thyme

1 medium lemon

10 strips bacon

Salt and pepper to taste

1 tbsp. grain mustard.

Directions

1. Oven preheats to 500°F.

2. Season chicken with salt and pepper, then lemon stuff, and thyme. Cover bacon with salt and pepper over bird skin, and season bacon.

3. Place the bird in a roasting saucepan and place it in the oven for 15 minutes. Reduce the temperature to 350°F and bake for 40-50 minutes.

4. Remove the bird and put it in foil.

5. Drizzle the juices into a pan and bring to a boil.

6. Add mustard, stir in, and slightly reduce to pan liquids. Then, use an immersion blender to blend sauce into the pan.

7. Serve with gravy on chicken.

Nutrition

Calories 376 | Fats: 29.8g | Carbs: 6.1g | Protein: 24.5g.

CHICKEN WITH MEDITERRANEAN SAUCE

Prep time: 4 min

Cook time: 16 min

Servings: 06

Ingredients

1 stick butter

½ pounds of chicken breasts

2 tsp. red wine vinegar

½ tbsp. olive oil

⅓ cup fresh Italian parsley, chopped

1 tbsp. green garlic

2 tbsp. red onions

Flaky sea salt and ground black pepper, to taste.

Directions

1. In a cast-iron skillet, heat the oil over a moderate flame. Sear the chicken for 10 to 12 minutes or until no longer pink. Season with salt and black pepper.

2. Add in the melted butter and continue to cook until heated through. Stir in the green garlic, onion, and Italian parsley; let it cook for 3 to 4 minutes more.

3. Mix in red wine vinegar and pull away from the heat.

Nutrition

Calories 411 kcal | Fat: 21g | Carbs: 19.7g | Protein: 36g.

TURKEY-PEPPER MIX

Prep time: 20 min

Cook time: 0 min

Servings: 01

Ingredients

1-pound turkey tenderloin

1 tsp. salt, divided

2 tbsp. extra-virgin olive oil

½ sweet onion, sliced

1 red bell pepper, cut into strips

1 yellow bell pepper, cut into strips

½ tsp. Italian seasoning

¼ tsp. ground black pepper

2 tsp. red wine vinegar

1 (14-ounces) can crush tomatoes.

Directions

1. Sprinkle ½ teaspoon salt on your turkey. Pour 1 tablespoon oil into the pan and heat it. Add the turkey steaks and cook for 1-3 minutes per side. Set aside.

2. Put the onion, bell peppers, and the remaining salt to the pan and cook for 7 minutes, stirring all the time. Sprinkle with Italian seasoning and add black pepper. Cook for 30 seconds. Add the tomatoes and vinegar and fry the mix for about 20 seconds.

3. Return the turkey to the pan and pour the sauce over it. Simmer for 2-3 minutes. Top with chopped parsley and basil.

Nutrition

Calories 230 kcal | Fat: 8g | Carbs: 6.8g | Protein: 30g.

CHICKEN PAN WITH VEGGIES & PESTO

Prep time: 10 min

Cook time: 20 min

Servings: 04

Ingredients

2 tbsp. olive oil

1-pound chicken thighs

¾ cup oil-packed sun-dried tomatoes

1-pound asparagus ends

¼ cup basil pesto

1 cup cherry tomatoes, red and yellow.

Directions

1. Cook olive oil in a frying pan over medium-high heat.

2. Put salt on the chicken slices and the put into a skillet, add the sun-dried tomatoes and fry for 5-10 minutes. Remove the chicken slices and season with salt. Add asparagus to the skillet. Cook for additional 5-10 minutes.

3. Position the chicken back in the skillet, pour in the pesto and whisk. Fry for 1-2 minutes. Remove from the heat. Add the halved cherry tomatoes and pesto. Stir well and serve.

Nutrition

Calories 423 kcal | Fat: 32g | Carbs: 8.9g | Protein: 2g.

CHICKEN QUESADILLAS

Prep time: 10 min

Cook time: 15 min

Servings: 02

Ingredients

1½ cups Mozzarella cheese, shredded

1½ cups Cheddar cheese, shredded

1 cup chicken, cooked and shredded

1 bell pepper, sliced

¼ cup tomato, diced

⅛ cup green onion

1 tbsp. extra-virgin olive oil

Directions

1. Preheat the oven to 400°F. Use parchment paper to cover a pizza pan.

2. Combine your cheeses and bake the cheese shell for about 5 minutes.

3. Put the chicken on one half of the cheese shell. Add peppers, tomatoes, green onion and fold your shell in half over the fillings.

4. Return your folded cheese shell to the oven again for 4-5 minutes.

Nutrition

Calories 244 kcal | Fat: 40.5g | Carbs: 6.1g. |Protein: 52.7g.

CREAMY GARLIC CHICKEN

Prep time: 5 min

Cook time: 15 min

Servings: 04

Ingredients

4 chicken breasts

1 tsp. garlic powder

1 tsp. paprika

2 tbsp. butter

1 tsp. salt

1 cup heavy cream

½ cup sun-dried tomatoes

2 cloves garlic

1 cup spinach.

Directions

1. Blend the paprika, garlic powder, and salt and sprinkle over both sides of the chicken.

2. Melt the butter in a frying pan (choose medium heat). Add the chicken breast and fry for 5 minutes each side. Set aside.

3. Add the heavy cream, sun-dried tomatoes, and garlic to the pan and whisk well to combine. Cook for 2 minutes. Add spinach and sauté for an additional 3 minutes.

4. Return the chicken to the pan and cover with the sauce

Nutrition

Calories 280 kcal | Fat: 26g | Carbs: 8g | Protein: 4g.

EASY ONE-PAN GROUND BEEF AND GREEN BEANS

Prep time: 13 min

Cook time: 6 min

Servings: 02

Ingredients

10 oz. (18-20) ground beef

9 oz. green beans

Pepper and salt, to taste

2 tbsp. sour cream

3½ oz. butter.

Directions

1. Rinse green beans, then trim the ends off each side.

2. Place half of the butter to a pan (that can fit the ground green beans and beef) over high heat.

3. Once hot, stir in the ground beef and season. Cook the beef until it's almost done.

4. Set heat on the pan to medium. Cook rest of butter and green beans to the pan for five minutes. Stir the ground beef and green beans rarely.

5. Season the green beans, with the pan drippings.

Nutrition

Calories 787.5 kcal | Fats: 71.75g | Carbs: 0.6g | Protein: 27.5g.

SHEET PAN BURGERS

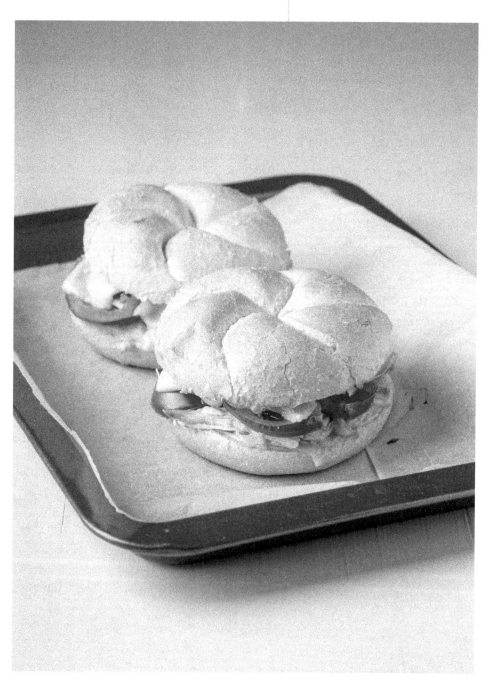

Ingredients

24 oz. ground beef

Sea salt & pepper, to taste

½ tsp. garlic powder

6 slices bacon, halved

1 med. onion, sliced into ¼ rounds

2 jalapeños, seeded & sliced

4 slices pepper jack cheese

¼ cup mayonnaise

1 tbsp. chili sauce

½ tsp. Worcestershire sauce

8 lg. leaves of Boston or butter lettuce

8 dill pickle chips.

Directions

1. Prep the oven to 425°F and line a baking sheet with non-stick foil.

2. Mix the salt, pepper, and garlic into the ground beef and form 4 patties out of it.

3. Line the burgers, bacon slices, jalapeño slices, and onion rounds onto the baking sheet and bake for about 18 minutes.

4. Garnish each patty with a piece of cheese and set the oven to boil.

5. Broil for 2 minutes, then remove the pan from the oven.

6. Serve one patty with 3 pieces of bacon, jalapeño slices, onion rounds, and desired amount of sauce with 2 pickle chips and 2 pieces of lettuce.

Nutrition

Calories 608 kcal | Fat: 46g | Carbs: 5g | Protein: 42g.

RICH AND EASY PORK RAGOUT

Prep time: 15 min

Cook time: 45 min

Servings: 04

Ingredients

1 tsp. lard, melted at room temperature

¾-pound pork butt

1 red bell pepper

1 poblano pepper

2 cloves garlic

½ cup leeks

½ tsp. mustard seeds

¼ tsp. ground allspice

¼ tsp. celery seeds

1 cup roasted vegetable broth

2 vine-ripe tomatoes, pureed.

Directions

1. Melt the lard in a stockpot over moderate heat. Once hot, cook the pork cubes for 4 to 6 minutes, occasionally stirring to ensure even cooking.

2. Then, stir in the vegetables and continue cooking until they are tender and fragrant. Add in the salt, black pepper, mustard seeds, allspice, celery seeds, roasted vegetable broth, and tomatoes.

3. Reduce the heat to simmer. Let it simmer for 30 minutes longer or until everything is heated through. Ladle into individual bowls and serve hot.

Nutrition

Calories 389 kcal | Fat 24.3g | Carbs: 5.4g | Protein: 22.7g.

MEXICAN CASSEROLE

Prep time: 8 min

Cook time: 50 min

Servings: 06

Ingredients

1-pound lean ground beef

2 cups salsa

1 (16 oz.) can chili beans, drained

3 cups tortilla chips, crushed

2 cups sour cream

1 (2 oz.) can slice black olives, drained

½ cup chopped green onion

½ cup chopped fresh tomato

2 cups shredded Cheddar cheese.

Directions

1. Prep oven to 350°F.

2. In a big wok over medium heat, cook the meat so that it is no longer pink. Add the sauce, reduce the heat and simmer for 20 minutes or until the liquid is absorbed. Add beans and heat.

3. Sprinkle a 9x13 baking dish with oil spray. Pour the chopped tortillas into the pan and then place the meat mixture on it.

4. Pour sour cream over meat and sprinkle with olives, green onions, and tomatoes. Top with cheddar cheese.

5. Bake in preheated oven for 30 minutes or until hot and bubbly.

Nutrition

Calories 597 kcal | Fat: 43.7g | Carbs: 32.8g | Protein: 31.7g.

PULLED PORK, MINT & CHEESE

Prep time: 20 min
Cook time: 15 min
Servings: 02

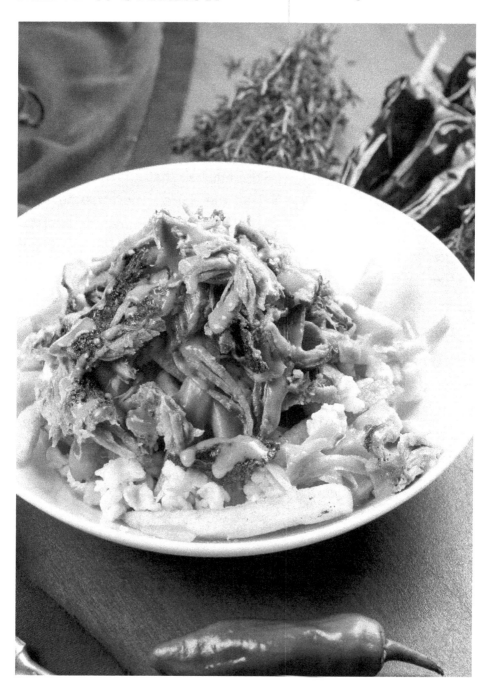

Ingredients

1 tsp. lard, melted at room temperature

¾ pork Boston butt, sliced

2 garlic cloves, pressed

½ tsp. red pepper flakes, crushed

½ tsp. black peppercorns, freshly cracked

Sea salt, to taste

2 bell peppers, deveined and sliced

1 tbsp. fresh mint leave snipped

4 tbsp. cream cheese.

Directions

1. Melt the lard in a cast-iron skillet over a moderate flame. Once hot, brown the pork for 2 minutes per side until caramelized and crispy on the edges.

2. Reduce the temperature to medium-low and continue cooking another 4 minutes, turning over periodically. Shred the pork with two forks and return to the skillet.

3. Add the garlic, red pepper, black peppercorns, salt, and bell pepper and continue cooking for a further 2 minutes or until the peppers are just tender and fragrant.

4. Serve with fresh mint and a dollop of cream cheese. Enjoy!

Nutrition

Calories 370 kcal | Fat: 21.9g | Carbs: 16g | Protein: 34.9g.

PORK

CHOP

Prep time: 10 min

Cook time: 30 min

Servings: 02

Ingredients

12 pork chops,
boneless, thin cut
2 cups baby spinach
4 cloves of garlic
12 slices Provolone
cheese.

Directions

1. Prep oven to a temperature of 350°F.
2. Pound the garlic cloves using a garlic press. The cloves should go through the press and into a small bowl.
3. Spread the garlic that you have made onto one side of the pork chops.
4. Flip half a dozen chops while making sure the garlic side is down. You should do this on a baking sheet that is rimmed.
5. Divide your spinach between the half dozen chops.
6. Fold cheese slices in half. Situate them on top of spinach.
7. Position the second pork chop on top of the first set, but this time make sure that the garlic side is up.
8. Bake for 20 minutes.
9. Cover each chop with another piece of cheese.
10. Bake another 15 minutes.

11. Your meat meter should be at 160°F when you check with a thermometer.

12. Serve hot and enjoy!

Nutrition

Calories 436 kcal | Fat: 25g | Carbs: 9.2g | Protein: 47g.

CAULIFLOWER CASSEROLE

Prep time: 15 min

Cook time: 35 min

Servings: 04

Ingredients

1 large head cauliflower

2 tbsp. butter

2 oz. cream cheese

1¼ cup sharp cheddar cheese

1 cup heavy cream

¼ cup scallion.

Directions

1. Preheat the oven to 350°F.
2. In a huge pan of boiling water, mix the cauliflower florets and cook for about 2 minutes.
3. Drain cauliflower and keep aside.
4. For cheese sauce: in a medium pan, add butter over medium-low heat and cook until just melted.
5. Add cream cheese, 1 cup of cheddar cheese, heavy cream, salt and black pepper and cook until melted and smooth, stirring continuously.
6. Pull away from heat and keep aside to cool slightly.
7. In a baking dish, place cauliflower florets, cheese sauce, and 3 tablespoons of scallion and stir to combine well.
8. Sprinkle with remaining cheddar cheese and scallion.
9. Bake for about 30 minutes.

10. Remove the casserole dish from oven and set aside for about 5-10 minutes before serving.

11. Cut into 4 equal-sized portions and serve.

Nutrition

Calories 365 kcal | Fat: 14g | Carbs: 5.6g | Protein: 12g.

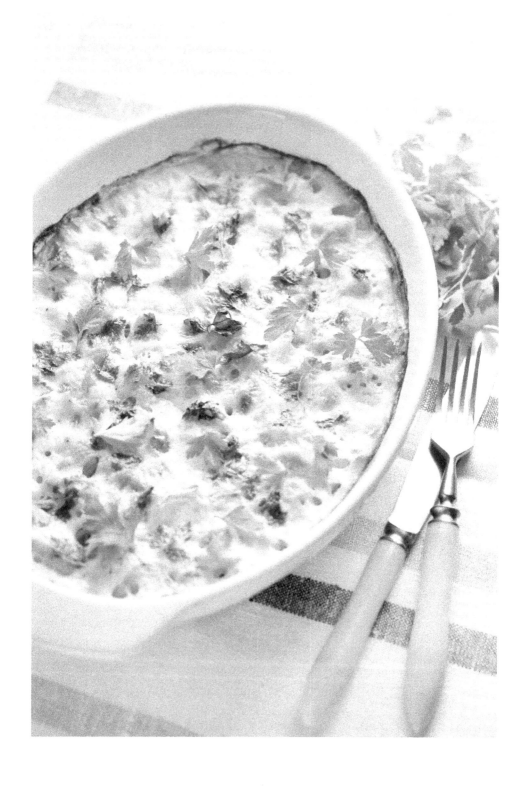

RICOTTA & BEEF STUFFED ZUCCHINI

Prep time: 15 min

Cook time: 30 min

Servings: 04

Ingredients

4 medium zucchini

1/2 lb. ground beef

2 large eggs

¾ cup part-skim Ricotta cheese

½ cup Parmesan cheese, grated

1 garlic clove,, minced

1 tbsp. dried basil

1 tbsp. fresh parsley, chopped

¾ tsp. salt

¼ tsp. ground black pepper

Extra virgin olive oil for drizzling.

Directions

1. Preheat the oven to 450°F. Line a baking sheet with parchment paper.

2. Half zucchini lengthwise. Remove the pulp from the center with a teaspoon, keeping the skin intact.

3. In a large bowl combine finely chopped zucchini pulp with all of the other ingredients and mix well. Divide the mixture between 8 zucchini halves.

4. Arrange stuffed zucchini on baking sheet, sprinkle with a little salt and drizzle with olive oil. Bake for 25-30 minutes until zucchini is tender and filling is beginning to brown. Serve hot.

Nutrition

Calories 322 kcal | Fat 20g | Carbs: 8g | Protein: 14g.

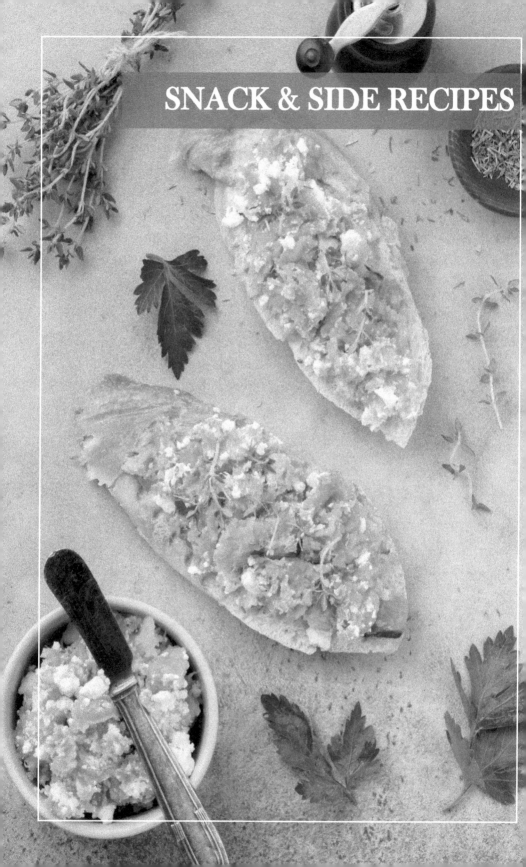

CAULIFLOWER BREADSTICKS

Prep time: 10 min

Cook time: 1h 35min

Servings: 04

Ingredients

4 eggs

4 cups of cauliflower riced

2 cups mozzarella cheese

4 cloves minced garlic

3 tsp. oregano.

Directions

1. Ready oven to 425°F. Line baking sheet by using parchment paper.

2. Situate cauliflower in a food processor or blender until finely chopped or when it resembles rice.

3. Put it in a covered bowl and microwave for just 10 minutes. Allow it to cool and if it's a little wet, make sure to drain it first before adding eggs, oregano, garlic, salt, pepper, and mozzarella. Mix them well.

4. Start separating the mixture into individual sticks – or really, just about any form you want.

5. Bake for 25 minutes. Pull out form the oven and sprinkle some more mozzarella on top while still hot. Put it back in the oven for just 5 minutes so that the cheese melts.

Nutrition

Calories 99 kcal | Fat: 19g | Carbs: 4g | Protein: 13g.

SPINACH IN CHEESE ENVELOPES

Prep time: 15 min

Cook time: 30 min

Servings: 08

Ingredients

3 cup cream cheese

1½ cup coconut flour

3 egg yolks

2 eggs

½ cup cheddar cheese

2 cups steamed spinach

¼ tsp. salt

½ tsp. pepper

¼ c. chopped onion.

Directions

1. Place cream cheese in a mixing bowl then whisks until soft and fluffy.

2. Add egg yolks to the mixing bowl then continue whisking until incorporated.

3. Stir in coconut flour to the cheese mixture then mix until becoming a soft dough.

4. Place the dough on a flat surface then roll until thin.

5. Cut the thin dough into 8 squares then keep.

6. Crash the eggs then place in a bowl. Season with salt, pepper, and grated cheese then mix well.

7. Add chopped spinach and onion to the egg mixture then stir until combined.

8. Put spinach filling on a square dough then fold until becoming an envelope.

9. Repeat with the remaining spinach filling and dough. Glue with water.

10. Preheat an Air Fryer to 425°F. Arrange the spinach envelopes in the Air Fryer

then cook for 12 minutes or until lightly golden brown.

11. Remove from the Air Fryer then serve warm. Enjoy!

Nutrition

Calories 365 kcal | Fat: 34g | Protein: 10g.

MOZZARELLA CHEESE POCKETS

Ingredients

1 large egg

8 pcs. of mozzarella cheese sticks

1¾ cup mozzarella cheese

¾ cup almond flour

1 oz. cream cheese

½ cup of crushed pork rinds.

Directions

1. Start by grating the mozzarella cheese.
2. Scourge the almond flour, mozzarella, and the cream cheese. Microwave them for 3 seconds until you get that delicious gooey mixture.
3. Put in a large egg and mix the whole thing together. You should get a nice thick batch of dough.
4. Put the dough in between two wax papers and roll it around until you get a semi-rectangular shape
5. Cut them into smaller rectangle pieces and wrap them around the cheese sticks. Mold it depending on the shape you want.
6. Roll the stick onto crushed pork rinds. Bake for 20 to 25 minutes at 400°F.

Nutrition

Calories 272 kcal | Fat: 22g | Carbs: 11g | Protein: 17g.

CATFISH BITES

Prep time: 12 min

Cook time: 16 min

Servings: 06

Ingredients

1-pound catfish fillet

1 tsp. minced garlic

1 large egg

½ onion, diced

1 tbsp. butter, melted

1 tsp. turmeric

1 tsp. ground thyme

1 tsp. ground coriander

¼ tsp. ground nutmeg

1 tsp. flax seeds.

Directions

1. Cut the catfish fillet into 6 bites.

2. Sprinkle the fish bites with the minced garlic. Stir it.

3. Then add diced onion, turmeric, ground thyme, ground coriander, ground nutmeg, and flax seeds. Mix the catfish bites gently.

4. Prep air fryer to 360°F.

5. Spray the catfish bites with the melted butter. Then freeze them.

6. Put the catfish bites in the air fryer basket and cook for 16 minutes.

7. When the dish is cooked – chill it. Enjoy!

Nutrition

Calories 140 kcal | Protein: 13.1g | Fats: 8.7g | Carbs: 4.2g.

KETO EGGS & PORK CUPS

Prep time: 15 min

Cook time: 40 min

Servings: 06

Ingredients

Cooking spray, for pan

2 lb. ground pork

2 cloves garlic, minced

½ tsp. paprika

1 tbsp. freshly chopped thyme

½ tsp. ground cumin

1 tsp. salt

Freshly ground black pepper, to taste

2½ cup chopped fresh spinach

1 cup shredded white cheddar

12 eggs

1 tbsp. freshly chopped chives.

Directions

1. Preheat oven to 400°F.

2. In a large bowl, combine ground pork, garlic, paprika, thyme, cumin, salt and pepper.

3. Prep 12 cups muffin tin with cooking spray. Add a small handful of pork to each muffin tin well then press up the sides to create a cup.

4. Divide spinach and cheese evenly between cups. Crack an egg on top of each cup and season with salt and pepper. Bake until eggs are set, and pork is cooked through, about 25 minutes.

5. Garnish with chives and serve. Enjoy!

Nutrition

Calories 385 kcal | Fat: 39g | Carbs: 3g |Protein: 16g.

ZUCCHINI MUFFINS

Prep time: 15 min
Cook time: 15 min
Servings: 04

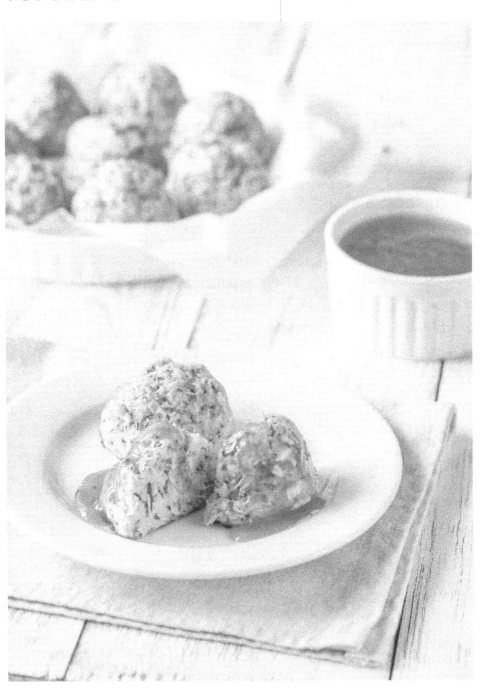

Ingredients

4 organic eggs

¼ cup unsalted butter, melted

¼ cup water

⅓ cup coconut flour

½ tsp. organic baking powder

¼ tsp. salt

1½ cups zucchini, grated

½ cup Parmesan cheese, shredded

1 tbsp. fresh oregano, minced

1 tbsp. fresh thyme, minced

¼ cup cheddar cheese, grated.

Directions

1. Preheat the oven to 400ºF.
2. Lightly, grease 8 muffin tins.
3. Add eggs, butter, and water in a mixing bowl and beat until well combined.
4. Add the flour, baking powder, and salt, and mix well.
5. Add remaining ingredients except for cheddar and mix until just combined.
6. Place the mixture into prepared muffin cups evenly.
7. Bake for approximately 13–15 minutes or until top of muffins become golden-brown.
8. Remove the muffin tin from oven and situate onto a wire rack for 10 minutes.
9. Carefully invert the muffins onto a platter and serve warm.

Nutrition

Calories 287 kcal | Fat: 23g | Carbs: 8.7g | Protein: 13.2g.

KETO GARLIC BREAD

Prep time: 5 min

Cook time: 30 min

Servings: 04

Ingredients

1 cup Mozzarella cheese, shredded

½ cup almond flour

2 tbsp. cream cheese

1 tbsp. garlic powder

1 tsp. baking powder

Salt, to taste

1 large egg

1 tbsp. butter, melted

1 clove garlic, minced

1 tbsp. freshly chopped parsley

1 tbsp. Parmesan cheese, freshly grated

Marinara, warmed, for serving.

Directions

1. Preheat oven to 400°F and line a large baking sheet with parchment paper.

2. In a medium, microwave-safe bowl, add mozzarella, almond flour, cream cheese, garlic powder, baking powder, and a large pinch of salt. Microwave on high until cheeses are melted, about 1 minute. Stir in egg. Shape dough into a baking sheet.

3. In a small bowl, mix melted butter with garlic, parsley, and Parmesan. Brush mixture over top of bread. Bake until golden, 15 to 17 minutes. Slice and serve with marinara sauce for dipping.

Nutrition

Calories 250 kcal | Fat: 20g | Carbs: 7g | Protein: 13g.

BRIE CHEESE
FAT BOMBS

Prep time: 45 min

Cook time: 3 min

Servings: 06

Ingredients

2 oz. cream cheese, full fat

½ cup Brie cheese, chopped

1 white onion, diced

1 tsp. paprika

6 lettuce leaves

¼ cup butter, unsalted

1 tbsp. ghee

1 clove garlic, minced

Salt and pepper, to taste.

Directions

1. Mix the cream cheese and the butter in a food processor and transfer to a bowl. When finished mix in the Brie.

2. Add the onion and the garlic in a pan and cook for approximately 3 minutes over medium heat with the ghee. Let cool.

3. Once cooled, combine with the cheese and the butter mixture. Season with the spices and mix.

4. Refrigerate for a minimum of 30 minutes. Make 6 fat bombs out of the mixture.

5. Serve on lettuce leaves.

Nutrition

Calories 158 kcal | Protein: 3.3g | Fat: 16.2g | Carbs: 2g.

SAVORY FAT BOMBS

Prep time: 1 h

Cook time: 5 min

Servings: 06

Ingredients

3.5 oz. cream cheese

¼ cup butter, cubed

2 large (2.1 oz.) slices of bacon

1 medium (0.5 oz) spring onion

1 clove garlic, crushed.

Directions

1. Add a cream cheese and butter to a bowl. Leave uncovered to soften at room temperature.

2. While that softens, set your bacon in a skillet on medium heat and cook until crisp. Allow it to cool then crumble into small pieces.

3. Add in your remaining ingredients to your cream cheese mixture and mix until fully combined.

4. Spoon small molds of your mixture onto a lined baking tray (about 2 tablespoons per mold). Then place to set in the freezer for about 30 minutes.

5. Set your Air Fryer to preheat to 350°F. Put in the Air Fryer basket with gap in between and cook for 5 minutes.

6. Cool to room temperature.

Nutrition

Calories 108 kcal | Protein: 2.1g | Fats: 11.7g | Carbs: 3.4g.

CHORIZO AND AVOCADO FAT BOMBS

Prep time: 45 min

Cook time: 8 min

Servings: 04

Ingredients

3.5 oz. Spanish Chorizo sausage, diced

¼ cup butter, unsalted

1 tbsp. lemon juice

Salt and cayenne pepper, to taste

2 large, hard-boiled eggs, diced

2 tbsp. mayonnaise

2 tbsp. chives, chopped

4 avocado halves, pitted.

Directions

1. Fry chorizo for 5 minutes in a hot pan. Set aside.

2. Combine all the ingredients in a mixing bowl and season with salt and cayenne pepper to taste. Mash together with a fork.

3. Refrigerate for approximately 30 minutes, and then fill each avocado half with ¼ of the mixture. Serve.

Nutrition

Calories 419 kcal | Protein: 11.4g | Fat: 38.9g | Carbs: 9.1g.

STUFFED ZUCCHINI

Prep time: 15 min

Cook time: 18 min

Servings: 08

Ingredients

4 medium zucchinis

1 cup red bell pepper

½ cup Kalamata olives

½ cup fresh tomatoes

1 tsp. garlic

1 tbsp. dried oregano

½ cup feta cheese, crumbled.

Directions

1. Preheat your oven to 350ºF. Grease a large baking sheet.

2. With a melon baller, spoon out the flesh of each zucchini half. Discard the flesh.

3. In a bowl, mix together the bell pepper, olives, tomatoes, garlic, oregano, salt, and black pepper.

4. Stuff each zucchini half with the veggie mixture evenly. Arrange zucchini halves onto the prepared baking sheet and bake for about 15 minutes.

5. Now, set the oven to broiler on high. Top each zucchini half with feta cheese and broil for about 3 minutes. Serve hot.

Nutrition

Calories 59 kcal | Fat: 3.2g | Carbs: 0.9g | Protein: 2.9g.

BROCCOLI WITH BELL PEPPERS

Prep time: 15 min

Cook time: 10 min

Servings: 06

Ingredients

2 tbsp. butter

2 garlic cloves, minced

1 large yellow onion, sliced

3 large red bell peppers

2 cups small broccoli florets

1 tbsp. low-sodium soy sauce

¼ cup homemade vegetable broth.

Directions

1. In a large wok, melt butter oil over medium heat and sauté the garlic for about 1 minute.

2. Add the vegetables and stir fry for about 5 minutes.

3. Stir in the broth and soy sauce and stir fry for about 4 minutes or until the desired doneness of the vegetables.

4. Stir in the black pepper and remove from the heat. Serve hot.

Nutrition

Calories 74 kcal | Fat: 4.1g | Carbs: 14g | Protein: 2.1g.

MUSHROOMS AND SPINACH

Prep time: 10 min

Cook time: 10 min

Servings: 04

Ingredients

10 oz. spinach leaves

14 oz. mushrooms

2 garlic cloves

½ cup fresh parsley

1 onion

4 tbsp. olive oil

2 tbsp. balsamic vinegar.

Directions

1. Heat a pan with the oil over medium-high heat, add the garlic and onion, stir, and cook for 4 minutes.

2. Add the mushrooms, stir, and cook for 3 minutes.

3. Add the spinach, stir, and cook for 3 minutes.

4. Add the vinegar, salt, and pepper, stir, and cook for 1 minute.

5. Add the parsley, stir, divide between plates, and serve.

Nutrition

Calories 200 kcal | Fat: 4g | Carbs: 7.6g | Protein: 13.5g.

BRUSSELS SPROUTS AND BACON

Prep time: 10 min

Cook time: 30 min

Servings: 04

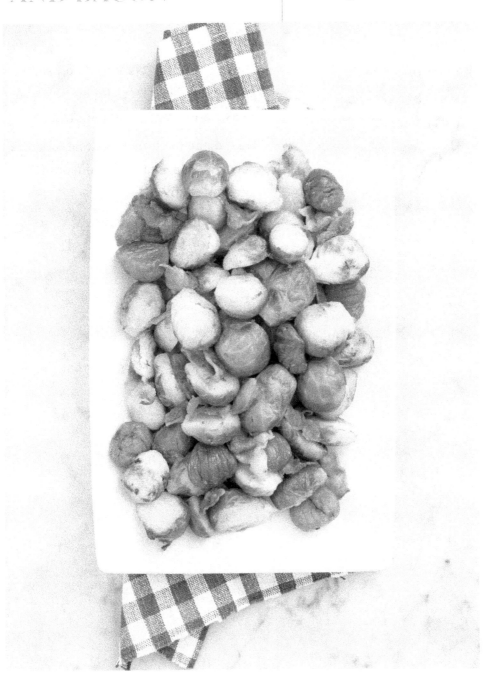

Ingredients

8 bacon strips, chopped

1-pound Brussels sprouts

A pinch of cumin

A pinch of red pepper, crushed

2 tbsp. extra virgin olive oil.

Directions

1. Toss Brussels sprouts with salt, pepper, cumin, red pepper, and oil to coat.

2. Spread the Brussels sprouts on a lined baking sheet, place in an oven at 375ºF, and bake for 30 minutes.

3. Heat a pan over medium heat, add the bacon pieces, and cook them until they become crispy.

4. Divide the baked Brussels sprouts on plates, top with bacon, and serve.

Nutrition

Calories 256 kcal | Fat 20g | Carbs: 7.6g | Protein: 32.2g.

INDIAN CAULIFLOWER RICE

Prep time: 5 min

Cook time: 20 min

Servings: 06

Ingredients

⅓ cup Ghee

2 garlic cloves, minced

½-inch Ginger, finely chopped

½ tsp ground turmeric

½ tsp. cumin seeds

1 tsp. coriander seeds

½ tsp. yellow mustard seeds

½ tsp. brown mustard seeds

26 oz. cauliflower processed into rice

2 tbsp. cilantro, chopped

Salt and black pepper, to taste.

Directions

1. Into a large non-stick frying pan over medium-high heat sauté the ghee, garlic and ginger and until fragrant.

2. Add all of the spices and sauté for 3 to 5 minutes.

3. Gently mix in half of the cauliflower rice and sauté for 3 minutes. Then stir in the remaining cauliflower rice.

4. Season with salt and pepper to taste and cook for another 8-10 minutes, mixing continuously, until softened.

5. Remove from heat and add the chopped cilantro. Serve hot.

Nutrition

Calories 224 kcal | Fat: 12g | Carbs: 7g | Protein: 4g.

AVOCADO SAUCE

Prep time: 10 min

Cook time: 0 min

Servings: 01

Ingredients

2 oz. pistachio nuts

1 tsp. salt

¼ cup lime juice

2 tbsp. garlic, minced

¼ cup water

⅔ cup olive oil

1 avocado

1 cup fresh parsley or cilantro.

Directions

1. Use a food processor or a blender to mix all of the ingredients together until they are smooth except the pistachio nuts and olive oil.

2. Add these at the end and mix well. If the mix is a bit thick add in a bit more oil or water.

Nutrition

Calories 490 kcal | Fat 50g | Carbs: 7.6g | Protein 5g.

BLUE CHEESE DRESSING

Prep time: 1 h

Cook time: 0 min

Servings: 01

Ingredients

2 tbsp. parsley, fresh

1 tsp. black pepper

1 tsp. salt

½ cup heavy whipping cream

½ cup mayonnaise

¾ cup greek yogurt

5 oz. blue cheese.

Directions

1. Break the blue cheese up into small chunks in a large bowl.

2. Stir in the heavy cream, mayonnaise, and yogurt.

3. Mix in the parsley, salt, and pepper and let the dressing sit for 1 hour, so the flavors mix well.

4. This dressing will be good in the refrigerator for three days.

Nutrition

Calories 477 kcal | Fat: 47g | Carbs: 12.5g | Protein: 10g.

SATAY SAUCE

Ingredients

1 can coconut cream

1 dry red pepper, seeds removed, chopped fine

1 clove garlic, minced

¼ cup gluten-free soy sauce

⅓ cup natural unsweetened peanut butter

Salt and pepper.

Directions

1. Place all ingredients in a small saucepan.

2. Bring the mixture to a boil.

3. Stir while heating to mix peanut butter with other ingredients as it melts.

4. After the mixture boils, turn down the heat to simmer on low heat for 5 to 10 minutes.

5. Remove from heat when the sauce is at the desired consistency.

6. Adjust seasoning to taste.

Nutrition

Calories 158 kcal | Fat: 13g | Carbs: 5g | Protein: 7g.

SALSA
DRESSING

Prep time: 1 h

Cook time: 0 min

Servings: 01

Ingredients

1 tbsp. garlic, minced

1 tsp. chili powder

3 tbsp. apple cider vinegar

2 tbsp. mayonnaise

2 tbsp. sour cream

¼ cup olive oil

½ cup salsa.

Directions

1. Mix all of the ingredients to a large bowl.

2. Pour into a glass jar and let the dressing chill in the refrigerator for at least one hour.

Nutrition

Calories 200 kcal | Fat: 21g | Carbs: 3.2g | Protein: 1g.

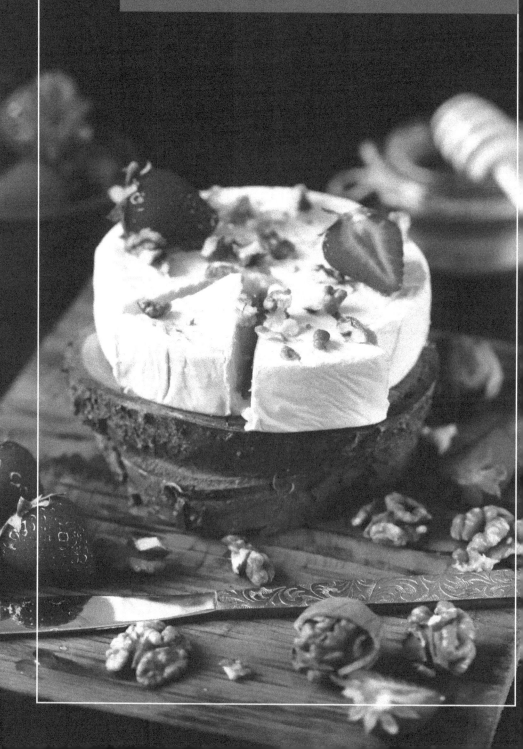

EASY PEANUT BUTTER CUPS

Prep time: 10 min
Cook time: 1h 35min
Servings: 12

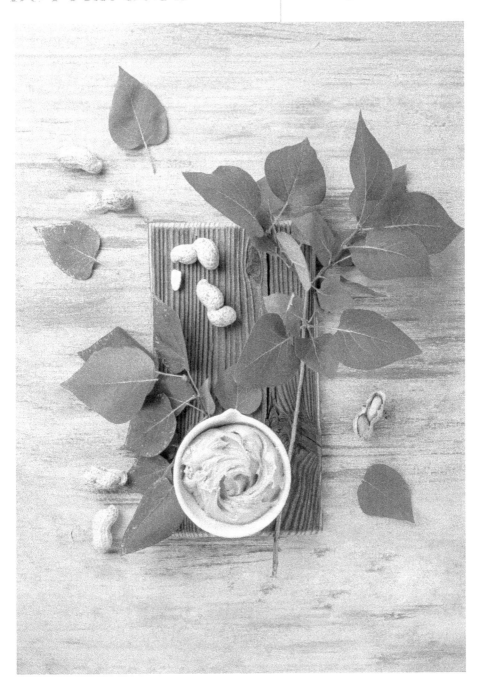

Ingredients

1/2 cup peanut butter

1/4 cup butter

3 oz. cacao butter, chopped

1/3 cup powdered swerve sweetener

1/2 tsp vanilla extract

4 oz. sugar-free dark chocolate.

Directions

1. Using low heat, melt the peanut butter, butter, and cacao butter in a saucepan. Stir them until thoroughly combined. Add the vanilla and sweetener until there are no more lumps.

2. Prepare muffin tin with parchment paper. Carefully place the mixture in the muffin cups. Refrigerate it until firm

3. Put chocolate in a bowl and set the bowl in boiling water. This is done to avoid direct contact with the heat. Stir the chocolate until completely melted.

4. Take the muffin out of the fridge and drizzle in the chocolate on top. Put it back again in the fridge to firm it up. This should take 15 minutes to finish.

5. Store and serve when needed.

Nutrition

Calories 200 kcal | Fat 19g | Carbs: 6g | Protein: 8g.

KETO MOCHA CHEESECAKE

Prep time: 10 min

Cook time: 0 min

Servings: 04

Ingredients

¾ cup heavy whipping cream

1 block of cream cheese (room temperature)

¼ cup unsweetened cocoa

¾ cup Swerve Confectioners sweetener

1 double shot of espresso.

Directions

1. Place the softened cream cheese in a bowl, and using a hand mixer, whip the cream cheese for 1 minute. Add espresso and continue mixing.

2. Add the sweetener, ¼ cup at a time and mix. Be sure to taste periodically, you may not need to use all the sweetener.

3. Add cocoa powder and mix until completely blended.

4. In a separate bowl, whip the cream until stiff peaks form.

5. Gently fold the whipped cream into the mocha mixture using a spatula. Place in individual serving dishes. Enjoy!

Nutrition

Calories 425 kcal | Protein: 6g | Fat: 33g | Carbs: 4.7g.

BLUEBERRY MUG CAKE

Prep time: 3 min

Cook time: 2 min

Servings: 02

Ingredients

2 tbsp. coconut flour

½ tsp. baking powder

25 grams fresh blueberries

1 large egg

2 tbsp. cream cheese

1 tbsp. butter

15 – 20 drips Liquid Stevia

¼ tsp. Himalayan Salt.

Directions

1. Add the butter and cream cheese to a mug and microwave for 20 seconds. Mix with a fork.

2. Add the baking powder, coconut flour and stevia and combine with a fork. Add the egg and combine.

3. Add the salt and fresh blueberries, and fold gently. Microwave for 90 seconds.

4. Eat right out of the mug or flip out onto a plate. For added flavor dust with powdered swerve.

Nutrition

Calories 345 kcal | Protein: 10g| Carbs: 8.7g | Fat: 29g.

LAVA

CAKE

Prep time: 10 min

Cook time: 0 min

Servings: 01

Ingredients

2 oz. unsweetened dark
chocolate

2 oz. unsalted butter

2 organic eggs

2 tbsp. powdered
Erythritol

1 tbsp. almond flour.

Directions

1. Preheat the oven to 350°F.

2. Grease 2 ramekins. In a microwave-safe bowl, add the chocolate and butter and microwave on High for about 2 minutes, stirring after every 30 seconds. Remove from the microwave and stir until smooth.

3. Place the eggs in a bowl and with a wire whisk, beat well. Add the chocolate mixture, Erythritol, and almond flour, and mix until well combined.

4. Divide the mixture into the prepared ramekins evenly. Bake for approximately 9 minutes or until the top is set.

5. Remove the ramekins from oven and set aside for about 1–2 minutes. Carefully, invert the cakes onto the serving plates and dust with extra powdered Erythritol.

Nutrition

Calories 478 kcal | Fat: 44g | Carbs: 8.5g | Protein: 9.6g.

LOW CARB
PECAN PIE

Prep time: 10 min

Cook time: 40 min

Servings: 12

Ingredients

For Crust

¼ cup butter

2 eggs

½ cup almond flour

¼ cup stevia

¼ tsp. salt

½ cup coconut flour

For Filling

¼ cup butter

2 eggs

½ cup sugar-free
caramel syrup

¼ cup granular stevia

2 tsp. vanilla extract

½ tsp. salt

1½ cup pecans,
chopped

Directions

To Make a Crust

1. In a medium microwavable bowl, melt butter for 30 seconds.

2. Stir in eggs, almond flour, stevia and salt.

3. Add sifted coconut flour and mix well.

4. Knead the dough with your hands for 1 minute, then shape it into a ball.

5. Roll out between wax paper to about ⅛-inch think and turn it into 9-inch pie pan.

6. Preheat the oven to 325°F.

To Make a Filling

7. In a medium microwavable bowl, melt butter for 30 seconds.

8. Beat melted butter, eggs, caramel syrup, stevia, vanilla extract and salt until well combined.

9. Stir in pecans.

10. Pour the mixture into the pie crust.

11. Bake for 35 to 40 minutes. The middle of the pie should not be set completely.

12. Let cool completely before serving.

Nutrition

Calories 250 kcal | Protein: 5.6g | Fat: 22g | Carbs: 4g.

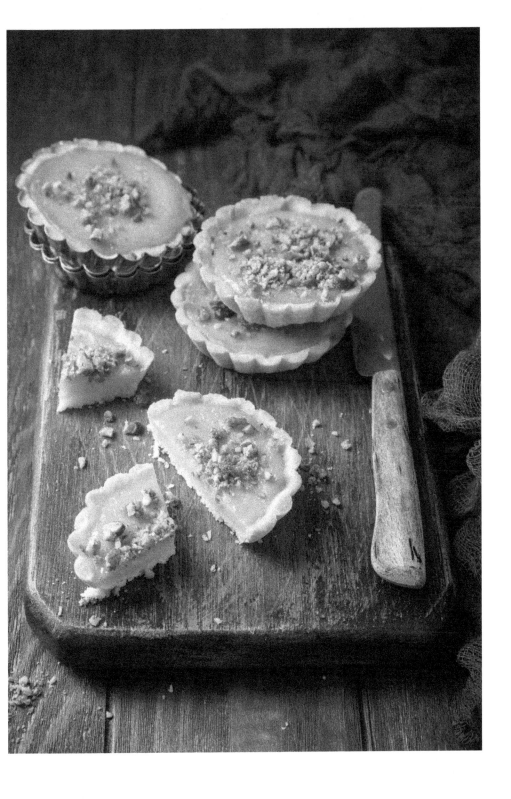

LOW CARB BUTTER COOKIES

Prep time: 10 min

Cook time: 10 min

Servings: 06

Ingredients

1 cup almond flour

¼ cup Confectioners Swerve

3 tbsp. salted butter (room temperature)

½ tsp. vanilla extract.

Directions

1. Preheat oven to 350°F.

2. Prepare a baking sheet lined with parchment paper or a nonstick baking mat.

3. In a mixing bowl, combine all ingredients, stirring thoroughly until resembling a dough. (it will look crumbly while you stir, then will form into a cohesive dough).

4. Form 1-inch balls, placing them on the baking sheet. There should be about 12 balls, separated from each other by about 2 inches.

5. Flatten each dough ball using a fork, then rotate 90 degrees and flatten again, forming a crisscross pattern.

6. Bake at 350°F until the cookie are golden around the edges, 8-10 minutes depending on the thickness of the cookies.

7. Let cool completely before removing them from the baking sheet, they cookies will be very soft when they first come out of the oven.

Nutrition

Calories 80 kcal | Protein: 2g | Fat: 8g | Carbs: 3.2g.

COCONUT & CHOCOLATE PUDDING

Prep time: 2 h 5 min

Cook time: 20 min

Servings: 06

Ingredients

2 egg yolks

14 oz. canned unsweetened coconut milk

1 tsp. vanilla extract

3 oz. sugar-free dark chocolate.

Directions

1. In a saucepan combine egg yolks and coconut milk and mix well. Place over medium low heat and let simmer while stirring for 10 minutes.

2. In a medium bowl add chocolate broken into small pieces and vanilla extract. Pour the coconut milk on top. Wait until the chocolate melts.

3. Whisk the batter and transfer into glasses.

4. Refrigerate for at least 2 hours before serving.

Nutrition

Calories 325 kcal | Protein: 5g| Carbs: 4.7g | Fat: 23g.

KETO ICE CREAM

Ingredients

2 (15-oz.) cans coconut milk

2 c. heavy cream

1/4 c. swerve confectioner's sweetener

1 tsp. pure vanilla extract

Pinch kosher salt.

Directions

1. Chill coconut milk in the fridge at least 3 hours, ideally overnight.

2. Make whipped coconut: Spoon coconut cream into a large bowl, leaving liquid in can, and use a hand mixer to beat coconut cream until very creamy. Set aside.

3. Make whipped cream: In a separate large bowl using a hand mixer (or in a bowl of a stand mixer), beat heavy cream until soft peaks form. Beat in sweetener and vanilla.

4. Fold whipped coconut into whipped cream, then transfer mixture into a loaf pan.

5. Freeze until solid, about 5 hours..

Nutrition

Calories 359 kcal | Protein: 11g| Carbs: 8g | Fat: 31g.

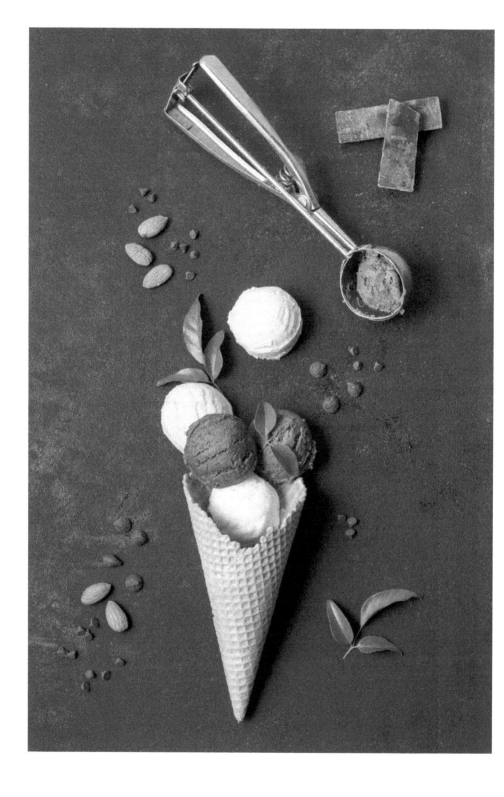

HOT CHOCOLATE

Prep time: 5 min

Cook time: 10 min

Servings: 01

Ingredients

2 tbsp. unsweetened cocoa powder, plus more for garnish

2 1/2 tsp. keto-friendly sugar, such as Swerve

1 1/4 c. water

1/4 c. heavy cream

1/4 tsp. pure vanilla extract

Whipped cream, for serving.

Directions

1. In a small saucepan over medium-low heat, whisk together cocoa, Swerve, and about 2 tablespoons water until smooth and dissolved. Increase heat to medium, add remaining water and cream, and whisk occasionally until hot.

2. Mix in vanilla, then pour into a mug. Serve with whipped cream and a dusting of cocoa powder...

Nutrition

Calories 118 kcal | Protein: 13g| Carbs: 11g | Fat: 21g.

The Ultimate Keto Diet Cookbook For Beginners | 113

PEANUT BUTTER COOKIES

Ingredients

1 1/2 c.smooth unsweetened peanut butter, melted (plus more for drizzling)

1 c. coconut flour

1/4 c. packed keto-friendly brown sugar

1 tsp. pure vanilla extract

Pinch salt

2 c. keto-friendly dark chocolate chips, melted

1 tbsp. coconut oil.

Directions

1. In a medium bowl, combine peanut butter, coconut flour, sugar, vanilla, and salt. Stir until smooth.

2. Line a baking sheet with parchment paper. Using a small cookie scoop, form mixture into rounds then press down lightly to flatten slightly and place on baking sheet. Freeze until firm, about 1 hour.

3. In a medium bowl, whisk together melted chocolate and coconut oil.

4. Using a fork, dip peanut butter rounds in chocolate until fully coated then return to baking sheet. Drizzle with more peanut butter then freeze until chocolate sets, about 10 minutes.

5. Serve cold. Store any leftovers in the freezer.

Nutrition

Calories 132 kcal | Protein: 7g| Carbs: 10g | Fat: 33g.

COOKIES TONIGHT!

Prep time: 10 min

Cook time: 35 min

Servings: 15

Ingredients

1/4 c. coconut oil

3 tbsp.

butter, softened

3 tbsp.granulated

Swerve sweetener

1/2 tsp.kosher salt

4 Large egg yolks

1 c.sugar-free dark

chocolate chips,

1 c. coconut flakes

3/4 c.chopped walnuts.

Directions

1. Preheat oven to 350° and line a baking sheet with parchment paper. In a large bowl stir together coconut oil, butter, sweetener, salt, and egg yolks. Mix in chocolate chips, coconut, and walnuts.

2. Drop batter by the spoonful onto prepared baking sheet and bake until golden, 14 to 16 minutes..

Nutrition

Calories 127 kcal | Protein: 3g| Carbs: 3g | Fat: 14g.

WALNUT SNOWBALLS

Prep time: 10 min

Cook time: 60 min

Servings: 15

Ingredients

1/2 c. (1 stick) melted butter

1 Large egg

1/4 tsp liquid stevia

1/2 tsp. pure vanilla extract

1 c. walnuts

1/2 c. coconut flour, plus 1 to 2 tbsp. more for rolling

1/2 c. confectioners Swerve, divided.

Directions

1. Preheat your oven to 300° and line a baking sheet with parchment paper. Combine melted butter, egg, stevia, and vanilla extract in a large bowl and set aside.

2. Add walnuts to a food processor and pulse until ground. Pour walnut flour into a medium bowl and add coconut flour and 1/4 cup Swerve and pulse until combined.

3. In 2 parts, add dry mixture to the wet and whisk to combine. At this point the dough should be soft but firm enough to form into balls by hand without it sticking to your palms.

4. Make 15 equal sized balls and arrange on prepared baking sheet. They will not spread in the oven.

5. Bake for 30 minutes.

6. Allow to cool for 5 minutes, and then roll the (still warm) balls in the remaining 1/4 cup Swerve.

7. Place them back on the parchment paper and allow to full cool, another 20 to 30 minutes, before eating

Nutrition

Calories 65 kcal | Protein: 2g| Carbs: 2g |
Fat: 9g.

CPSIA information can be obtained
at www.ICGtesting.com
Printed in the USA
BVHW090849140621
609525BV00002B/117